Ken Babal CN

Good Digestion

Your key to vibrant health

alive books
Vancouver
Canada

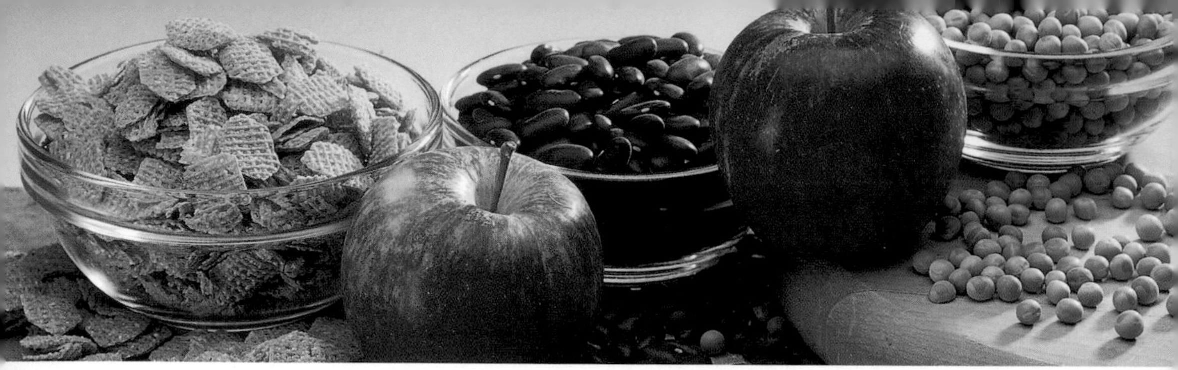

contents

Note: Conversions in this book (from imperial to metric) are not exact. They have been rounded to the nearest measurement for convenience. Exact measurements are given in imperial. The recipes in this book are by no means to be taken as therapeutic. They simply promote the philosophy of both the author and alive books in relation to whole foods, health and nutrition, while incorporating the practical advice given by the author in the first section of the book.

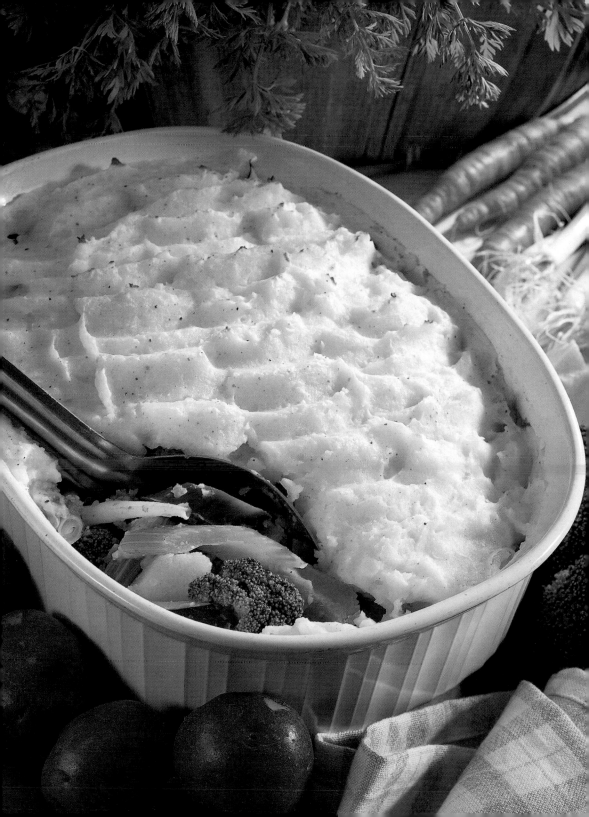

Phelan J., et al, "Coeliac disease, the abolition of gliadin toxicity by enzymes from Aspergillus niger." *Clin Sci Molec Med*, 1977, 53:35-43.

Misciagne, G., et al. "Diet, physical activity and gallstones–a population based, case control study in southern Italy." *Amer J Cln Nutr*, 1999; 69: 120-6.

Moerman, C., et al., "Dietary risk factors for clinically diagnosed gallstones in middle-aged men: a 25-year follow up study (the Zutphen study)." *Ann epidemiol*, 1994; 4: 248-54.

Treben, M., *Health Through God's Pharmacy*, Ennsthaler, 1986.

Ruddell, R., et al. "Effect of cimetidine and antacid on gastric bacterial flora", *The Lancet*, March 1980, 29:672-4.

Recker,R. "Calcium absorbtion and achlorhydria." *N Engl J Med*, 1985, 313: 70-73.

Belluzi, A., et tal. "Effect of an enteric-coated fish oil preparation on relapses in Crohn's disease", *N Eng J Med*, Vol. 334, No.24, June 13, 1996, pp. 1557-60

Bensoussan, A., et al. "Treatment of irritable bowel syndrome with Chinese herbal medicine", *JAMA*, Nov.11,1998, Vol 280, No.18 pp. 1585-89.

Willa, T., "Lactobacillus overgrowth for treatment of moniliary vulvovaginitis." *Lancet*, 1979;2: 482.

Hepner, G., et al., "Hypocholesterolemic effect of yogurt and milk." *Am J Cln Nutr*, 1979; 32; 19-24.

Beck, C., et al. "Beneficial effects of administration of Lactobacillus acidophilus in diarrheal and other intestinal disorders." *Am J Gastroenterol*, 1961; 35; 522.

Elmstahl, S., et al. "Fermented milk products are associated to ulcer disease. Results from a cross-sectional population study." *Euro J Clin Nutr*, 1998, 52: 668-674.

Gorbach, S., "The intestinal microflora and its colon cancer connection." *Infection*, 1982; 10: 379-384.

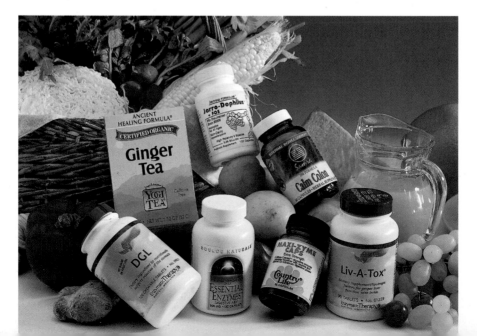

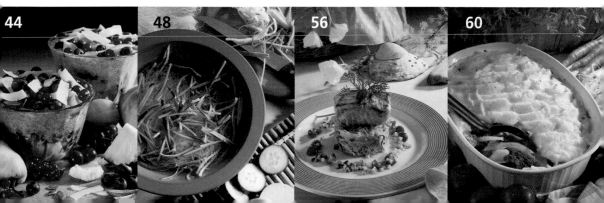

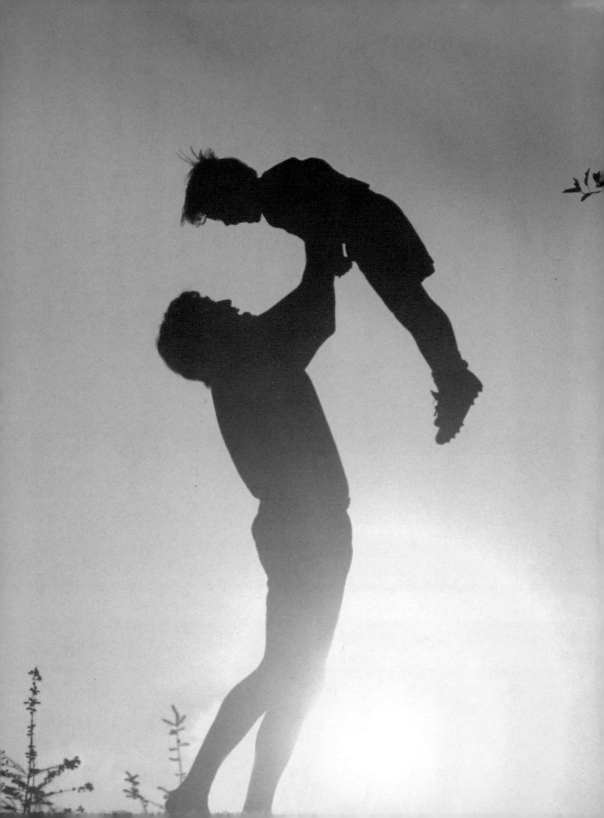

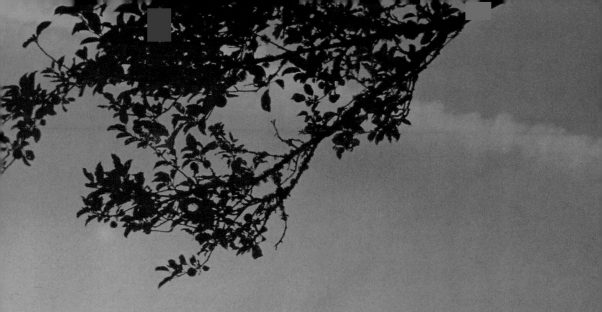

When a person maintains efficient digestion, a strong body chemistry results and all other systems benefit.

Digestion is the Key . . . .

Weight problems, eczema, acne, allergies, asthma, fatigue, constipation, anemia, gall stones, insomnia, infections, fungal problems, arthritis, osteoporosis, and certain types of cancer. What do these ailments have in common? All can be caused or worsened by poor digestion. The fact is, digestion is a key issue in any type of health problem and one the most important factors influencing your total well-being.

As a nutritionist, I know that if I can help a client resolve difficulties with digestion and elimination, we've achieved a great advantage in overcoming other health problems whether minor or severe. When a person maintains efficient digestion, a strong body chemistry is the result and all other systems begin to benefit. Also, if your digestion is functioning properly you have a better chance of maintaining well-being.

Digestion is a critical facet of nutrition. Nutrition is not just what we eat but what the cells of the body actually receive—and the cells only receive what is broken down through the process of digestion. Nutrients must traverse membrane barriers on a long voyage from the digestive tract into and out of the cells of the intestinal mucosa, vascular system and finally the cell membrane.

The fiber obtained from fruit and vegetables promotes good digestion.

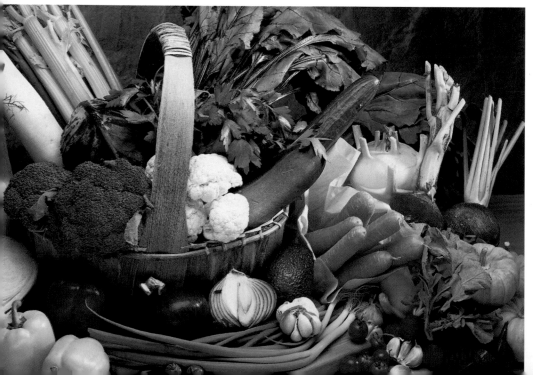

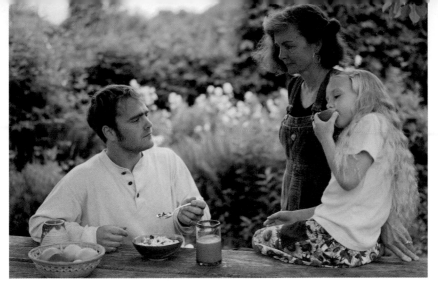

What the cells actually receive is rarely, if ever, optimum. To rephrase an old adage, we are not what we eat, but what we digest and absorb.

Eating in a relaxed, unhurried manner promotes good digestion.

The flip side of nutrient availability/absorption is how well we get rid of the waste products. *Cleanse* and *nourish* are the two factors in the health equation. Both processes occur within the gastrointestinal (GI) tract, which is where our fueling station and waste-management system is.

Digestive disturbances are very common and it is safe to say that most people experience some difficulty, especially those who do not enjoy good health. The prevalence of advertisements for antacids alone testifies to the extent of the problem. Stomach acid blockers are among the best-selling drugs of all time. Many of us accept indigestion as a normal part of eating when in fact we should be barely conscious of digestion. Gas, heartburn, bloating, burping, bad breath, constipation, diarrhea and general discomfort or fatigue after meals are common symptoms of poor digestion.

Although common, these symptoms should not be considered normal. They are distress signals that tell us the process is not going smoothly and we are not getting the full benefit of what we ate. They are also a warning that more serious problems may be down the road if we do not make the necessary dietary changes that prevent these occurrences. Big problems always start small and minor digestive disturbances can eventually lead to ulcers or conditions affecting other body systems not commonly associated with the GI tract.

When things go wrong in the intestinal tract, foreign substances normally excluded, such as toxins, partially digested food and micro-organisms, are absorbed and distributed throughout the system. This increased permeability of the intestinal mucosa, or "leaky gut" as it is sometimes called, is suspected of contributing to a number of systemic disorders including allergies, eczema, hives, autoimmune diseases, bowel diseases, and viral and bacteria infections. Sometimes the body can go for years with dietary abuse and faulty digestion with little overt sign of problems developing below. By the time they manifest, the connection is often missed.

You can expect noticeable improvements in digestion in a matter of days.

Digestion is the Key

I have seen many positive responses in people who learn the rules of digestion. Tracee, a woman I have known for many years, suffered from a duodenal ulcer that she says "had her by the throat" because of the extent it was interfering with her life. She had to buy Mylanta on sale because of her great dependency on antacids. Tracee began to change her life first by going on a short fast. She then stopped smoking and cut out fried foods and has never had a relapse in 20 years.

Warren, a young man diagnosed with ulcerative colitis, modified his diet and began taking supplements. He happily reports that his new program has definitely had a positive effect on his system. Laura, a 34 year old woman, says since taking an enzyme supplement she has better digestion and elimination and her skin does not break out as often.

Another client shed several pounds of fat without dieting just by taking apple cider vinegar with her meals. These are just several of hundreds of testimonials that have convinced me that people have the power to make great strides in their health by means of digestive support.

The good news is cells of the gastrointestinal lining turn over rapidly and healthy new cells are constantly replacing old, worn-out ones. Remarkably, every five days you have a new stomach lining. This means that if you are kind to your stomach and take advantage of natural remedies you can expect noticeable improvements in digestion and well-being in just a matter of days. You will then be on the road to vibrant health.

Journey Through the Gastrointestinal Tract . . .

The gastrointestinal tract is a twenty- to twenty-five-foot tube through the body beginning at the lips and ending at the anus. It acts like a conveyor belt taking food past several organs and through a series of processes to break it down and absorb it while getting rid of what we don't need. Protein is broken down into amino acids; carbohydrates (starch and complex sugars) into simple sugars; and fats into fatty acids and glycerol. Vitamins and minerals are also liberated. All of these simple molecules are able to pass through the walls of the intestine and into the bloodstream where ultimately they are used by cells for energy or as structural materials.

The mouth is an alkaline environment in which teeth and jaw muscles initiate the digestive process. Enzymes that digest starch are secreted here. Smell and taste make the saliva flow which eases passage of food toward the stomach, the first digestive organ.

The stomach also carries out a physical action of pummeling and squeezing the food into smaller fragments. Hydrochloric acid (HCl) is secreted which sterilizes the stomach contents and is required for efficient absorption of protein, fats and minerals. HCl, though strong enough to dissolve concrete, does not digest the stomach wall, which is normally protected by mucus secretions.

A series of wave-like muscular contractions pushes small amounts of food from the stomach into the duodenum, the first part of the intestine. Although a whole meal arrives in the stomach very quickly, it leaves in much smaller portions let through by the pyloric sphincter, a muscular ring leading to the intestine. Gastric acid is neutralized by bicarbonate, shifting the pH back to alkalinity.

Enzymes from the pancreas are then secreted to perform most of the

The gastrointestinal tract begins at the lips and ends at the anus.

9

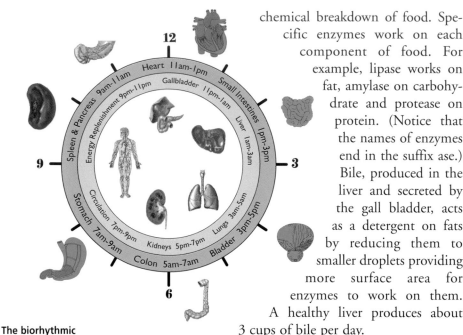

Heart 11am-1pm
Small Intestines 1pm-3pm
Gallbladder 11pm-1am
Liver 1am-3am
Energy Replenishment 9pm-11pm
Spleen & Pancreas 9am-11am
Lungs 3am-5am
Circulation 7pm-9pm
Bladder 3pm-5pm
Stomach 7am-9am
Kidneys 5pm-7pm
Colon 5am-7am
12
9
3
6

The biorhythmic clock shows when the organs involved in digestion are most active.

chemical breakdown of food. Specific enzymes work on each component of food. For example, lipase works on fat, amylase on carbohydrate and protease on protein. (Notice that the names of enzymes end in the suffix ase.) Bile, produced in the liver and secreted by the gall bladder, acts as a detergent on fats by reducing them to smaller droplets providing more surface area for enzymes to work on them. A healthy liver produces about 3 cups of bile per day.

The intestine is not a simple hose carrying food components from one end to the other. Nutrients have to be carried across the intestinal wall and what's left has to be squeezed dry. The muscle wall massages food onward in rhythmic contractions called peristalsis. It is pressed into contact with the intestinal wall which is lined with millions of tiny "fingers" called villi. If the intestine was just a smooth tube, the inner surface would measure about five square feet in area, but with the combined surfaces of all the villi, there is about 600 times as much area to absorb the food molecules more efficiently. Each of the villi has channels running through its core. These channels carry away the molecules of food into the bloodstream or, in the case of fats, the lymphatic system. It takes up to five hours to be turned into food the cells can use.

We've traveled about 20 feet by now. The last stage of our journey is the colon, the final five feet. Although most of the goodness from the food has been absorbed, there's one final food component—water. Remnants of food are still very wet when they reach this point. They will lose about two-thirds of their weight as water is squeezed out and absorbed. It has taken food about six hours to come this far. At this juncture is the appendix, an often troublesome blind alley open to any solid matter that can become infected if trapped. In animals, it contains plant-eating bacteria.

All that's left now is a mixture of fiber, bacteria and cells that we have to get rid of. Much of the residue is made up of plant fibers we can't easily digest. The solid matter in the colon, the feces, includes cells from the intestinal wall that have been rubbed off in the journey from the stomach.

Improved system functioning is partly attributed to the detoxification that occurs during a fast.

Fasting Broth

A vegetable broth provides potassium and other nutrients in an easily absorbed form. This is a good source of nourishment when the appetite is not good. During a fast, water normally obtained from foods can be replaced with broth, herb teas and juices.

2 large potatoes (unpeeled), chopped
2 celery stalks, chopped
1 large carrot (unpeeled), chopped
1 beet, chopped
1 teaspoon kelp powder or strip of kombu seaweed (optional)
6 cups distilled or spring water

Combine ingredients in a stainless steel, enameled or earthenware pot. Cover and bring to a boil; reduce heat and cook slowly for half an hour. Strain. Store in refrigerator. Warm the broth before drinking.

The intestine is populated with 100 trillion bacteria which account for about a third of the weight of the feces. These single-celled organisms are much undervalued inhabitants of the body. Many of these bacteria perform useful jobs in the body's cavities and surfaces. These "friendly" bacteria synthesize vitamins from food remnants, degrade toxins, prevent colonization of disease-causing micro-organisms, crowd out less beneficial bacteria, stimulate the immune system and produce short-chain fatty acids, an energy source for cells lining the colon.

Eventually, three times a day or only once every two or three days if we are constipated, the feces arrive at the rectum, the end of the journey. As we feel their arrival, a series of muscular contractions is set in motion to expel the feces and the job is complete.

Digestive Symptom Survey

The following symptom survey will help you determine how efficient your digestion is and which part of the gastrointestinal tract needs the most support. Under each section, score 0, 1, 2, 3 or as noted for each symptom depending on the severity and frequency. 0 = symptom not present 1 = mild/rare 2 = moderate/occasional 3 = severe/frequent

Section One

1. Burping_____
2. Hiccups_____
3. Fullness for extended time after meals_____
4. Bloating in stomach_____
5. Poor appetite_____
6. Stomach upsets easily_____
7. History of constipation_____
8. Known food allergies_____

Section Two

1. Abdominal cramps_____
2. Indigestion 1–3 hours after eating_____
3. Fatigue after eating_____
4. Lower bowel gas_____
5. Alternating constipation and diarrhea_____
6. Diarrhea_____
7. Fiber causes constipation_____
8. Mucus in stools_____
9. Stool poorly formed_____
10. Shiny stool_____
11. Foul-smelling stool_____
12. Dry flaky skin and/or dry brittle hair_____
13. Pain in left side under rib cage_____
14. Acne_____
15. Food allergies_____
16. Difficulty gaining weight_____

Section Three

1. Stomach pain_____
2. Stomach pain just before and/or after meals_____

3. Dependency on antacids/acid reducers_____
4. Chronic abdominal pain_____
5. Butterfly sensations in stomach_____
6. Stomach pain when emotionally upset_____
7. Sudden, acute indigestion_____
8. Relief of stomach pain by drinking cream/milk_____
9. Current ulcer   NO   YES(10) _____
10. Black stool (when not taking iron supplements/bismuth medications)   NO   YES(10) _____

Section Four
1. Frequent and recurrent infections (colds)_____
2. Bladder and kidney infections_____
3. Vaginal yeast infection_____
4. Abdominal cramps_____
5. Toe and fingernail fungus_____
6. Alternating diarrhea/constipation_____
7. Constipation_____
8. History of antibiotic use_____
9. Meat eater_____

Section Five
1. Intolerance to greasy foods_____
2. Yellow in whites of eyes_____
3. Light-colored stool_____
4. Hard stool_____
5. Sour or metallic taste in mouth_____
6. Bad breath_____
7. Body odor_____
8. Fatigue and sleepiness after eating_____
9. Frontal headaches after eating_____
10. Pain in right side under rib cage_____
11. Retain water_____
12. Dry skin/hair_____
13. Have or have had gallstones   NO   YES (3)_____
14. Have had jaundice or hepatitis   NO   YES (3)_____
15. High blood cholesterol with low HDL   NO   YES (10)_____
16. Known cholesterol level above 200   NO   YES (3)_____
17. Known triglyceride level above 115   NO   YES (3)_____

Results

Part One–Stomach (Low acidity)
0-4 low priority; 5-9 moderate priority; 10+ high priority
Supplements: herbal bitters, apple cider vinegar or betaine HCl

Part Two–Small Intestine/Pancreas
0-5 low priority; 6-9 moderate priority; 10+ high priority
Supplements: pancreatic or plant enzymes

Part Three–Stomach (Ulcers/Hyperacidity)
0-5 low priority; 6-9 moderate priority; 10+ high priority
Supplements: DGL (licorice), aloe vera juice/gel, slippery elm,
ginger, chlorophyll

Part Four–Colon
0-5 low priority; 6-9 moderate priority; 10+ high priority
Supplements: probiotics, fiber

Part Five–Liver/Pancreas
0-3 low priority; 4-6 moderate priority; 7+ high priority
Supplements: lipotropic supplement, choleretic herbs, fiber,
probiotics

10 Commandments for Good Digestion

1. Do not over-eat; smaller more frequent meals are best.
You are less likely to tax your digestive capability when you eat
modestly–and you'll be able to eat again sooner! Divide your
calories into three meals per day plus one or two snacks. Another
benefit is calories are less likely to be stored as fat when spaced
throughout the day. Do not go more than five hours without
eating unless fasting. When the blood sugar level falls we are
more likely to binge or reach for junk foods for a quick fix.

2. Keep meals as simple and as nutritious as possible.
For best results, combine only protein + vegetable or grain +
vegetable or eat a mono meal. Avoid fried foods.

3. Keep sweets to a minimum.
Sugars tend to ferment in the warm environment of the stomach.
Excessive amounts can cause gas, bloating and indigestion.

"Things sweet to
taste prove in
digestion sour."
–Shakespeare

14

4. Eat regular meals but only when truly hungry.
If you experience digestive discomfort, do not eat again until you feel completely comfortable with your last meal.

5. Do not consume ice-cold or sugary drinks with meals.
Drink only unchilled water, diluted juice or tea. They may be appropriate on a hot day, but consuming very cold drinks can shock the system (98.6° F) and cause fats to congeal in the stomach. Digestive herb teas are especially good to sip with or after meals. Liquids activate digestive juices but excessive amounts can also dilute them. Pay attention to your body's signals.

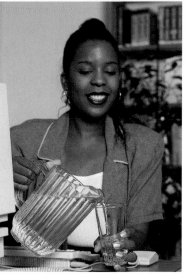

6. Relax–do not eat hurriedly.
Chew food well; don't eat a lot when feeling nervous or anxious. Stress causes the digestive system to shut down. It's only natural to eat until we're full. However, if we eat too hurriedly, we don't give the brain a chance to receive the signal that we're satisfied and we tend to overeat.

Drinking water should be unchilled so as not to shock the system.

7. Use caution with citrus fruits.
Citrus fruits (oranges, lemons and grapefruit) are cleansing to the system but can also be harsh. They do not combine well with starches (bread, crackers, potatoes, rice, etc). In general, fruit provides quick energy and helps with elimination but overuse can weaken digestion.

8. Obtain plenty of fiber in the diet.
Fiber is found in unrefined plant foods (whole grains, vegetables and fruit). The recommendation is 25 to 35 grams of dietary fiber a day except when acute bowel inflammation is present.

9. Limit or eliminate coffee (regular and decaf), alcohol and all drugs not prescribed by your doctor.

10. Take digestive enzymes with meals along with a multiple vitamin-mineral supplement.

Digestive Disorders . . . .

Celiac Disease

Celiac disease is a disorder in which damage to the surface of the small intestine is caused by the ingestion of food products that contain gluten or similar proteins that are present in wheat, rye, oats and barley. Such proteins are also present in hybrid grains such as triticale.

The following grains appear to be non-toxic to gluten-intolerant people but have never been specifically tested: amaranth, millet, quinoa, teff and buckwheat. Also acceptable to most celiac individuals are rice and corn.

The following products should definitely be avoided as all are forms of wheat: durum semolina, kamut and spelt. Celiac disease sufferers should avoid bulk foods since utensils containing particles of one food might be transferred to another bin with a different food item.

It is crucial that those with celiac disease carefully read food, drug and vitamin labels for hidden sources of gluten such as hydrolyzed vegetable protein (HVP), textured vegetable protein (TVP), hydrolyzed plant protein (HPP), malt, modified food starch, soy sauces which contain wheat and other prohibited

Amaranth, millet, quinoa, teff and buckwheat appear to be okay for gluten-intolerant people.

16

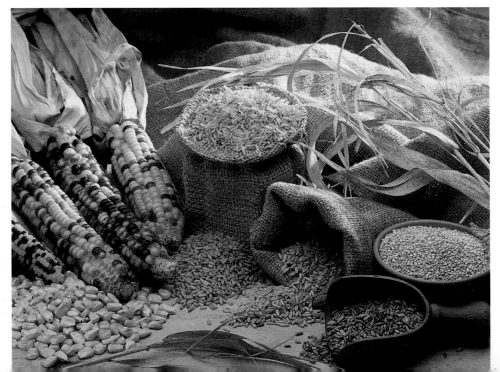

substances, grain vinegars, various binders, fillers, excipients and "natural flavorings."

Increased intestinal permeability is believed to be a contributor to celiac disease. (See "Leaky Gut Syndrome" on page 31). In test tube experiments, enzyme preparations are effective in rendering the components of gluten harmless to celiac patients. As yet, it has not been proven that taking enzyme supplements along with gluten-containing foods has the same effect. However, celiac patients may find such supplements helpful in reducing symptoms. Either pancreatin or plant enzymes can be used to enhance digestive function. Glutamine and gamma-oryzanol may be useful in healing the intestinal lining.

Constipation

Constipation is a decrease in the frequency of bowel movements accompanied by a difficult, prolonged effort in passing a hard stool. All too often doctors casually shrug off this condition, saying that it is completely normal for some people to only have two or three bowel movements per week.

Natural health practitioners tend to view this as incorrect and dangerous advice. Normally, it takes up to twenty hours for food to move through the digestive tract. Ideally, it should take twelve to eighteen hours.

Also, if you are straining or have any discomfort during elimination you are probably constipated.

The most common cause of constipation is a lack of fiber in the diet. However, other factors can contribute such as certain drugs, some iron or calcium supplements or hypothyroidism. For most people, increasing fiber and fluids solves the problem. Regular exercise is also very helpful. Two nutrients that have a natural laxative effect are vitamin C and magnesium. Reliance on stimulating laxatives causes dependency and loss of natural function.

Diarrhea

Diarrhea is an abnormally frequent passage of loose, watery stools. It is the body's way of getting rid of something it can't use. Often, diarrhea is caused by a bacterial infection such as food poisoning. Dietary diarrhea can be caused by certain foods such

The most common cause of constipation is a lack of fiber in the diet.

as citrus juice, figs, prunes, coffee or unripe fruit. Generally, loose stools are unabsorbed food caused by weak digestion or an imbalance in one's food selections. The non-digestible sugar alcohols sorbitol, mannitol and xylitol used as sugar substitutes in sugar-free candies and gum can cause diarrhea, gas and bloating.

Some natural remedies for diarrhea are blackberry tea, carob powder and a BRAT diet (banana, white rice, peeled apple and white toast). Other remedies are activated charcoal, bismuth, psyllium seed powder (creates bulk and helps to form a stool). Natural infection fighters for treating diarrhea caused by bacteria are goldenseal and *Citricidal* (grapefruit seed extract). All antibiotic treatments, whether natural or prescription, should be followed with probiotic supplementation. Probiotics help maintain a favorable balance of intestinal flora. Diarrhea, when not caused by a serious disorder, can usually be cured by taking one teaspoon of apple cider vinegar in water with meals and several times a day between meals.

Apple cider vinegar is a natural remedy for diarrhea.

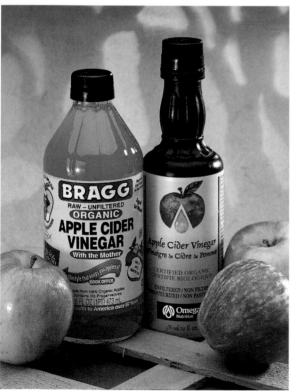

For persistent diarrhea, be sure to consult a physician. Chronic diarrhea can be a symptom of a more serious condition such as parasitic infection or inflammatory bowel disease and can be life-threatening in children or the elderly by causing dehydration and loss of electrolyte minerals.

Diverticulitis

Diverticulitis is an inflammation of small hernias or ruptures in the colon wall. The herniations resemble small pouches like that created by squeezing a balloon. The most common symptoms are pain and cramping usually in the lower left side of the abdomen. Diverticulitis results from excessive pressure in the colon and weakening of the wall. A low-fiber diet may be the main cause of diverticular disease.

A diet high in fiber and liquids will keep the colon healthy and prevent the chronic constipation that can lead to diverticulitis. *Lactobacillus acidophilus* will help to re-establish the natural bacteria in the bowels that exist to fend off illness. Silica helps rebuild connective tissue and reduce inflammation. And walking is a good exercise to activate bowel movements.

Gall Stones

The gall bladder is a small, pear-shaped sack that hangs between the lobes of the liver. It is the storage vessel for bile, a bitter, yellowish brown or brownish green liquid produced in the liver. When a meal containing fat enters the digestive tract, the gall bladder is stimulated to contract and secrete the bile into the small intestine.

Stones are sometimes formed in the gall bladder or bile duct, a passageway leading to the intestine. Common associations of gall stone patients are that they are usually women who are "fair, fat, forty and fertile." With age, the incidence tends to even out between men and women.

Gall stones consist of cholesterol, calcium and pigment. The most common type of stone (about 80 percent) is composed predominantly of cholesterol. These stones represent a type of cholesterol abnormality similar to the plaque that accumulates in arteries.

Stones begin to form when cholesterol, a normal component of bile, is over-secreted into the bile due to an impairment in liver function. When the ability of the bile acids to keep the cholesterol in solution is exceeded, cholesterol precipitates out of the bile, crystalizes and aggregates to form a stone.

Symptoms of gall bladder distress commonly occur several hours after a meal containing fat. They may include nausea, indigestion, vomiting and pain on the right side that radiates to the back or shoulder. Many people are without symptoms until a stone passes through the gall bladder and bile duct, producing debilitating pain. Pain is also felt when a stone impacts into the duct system and the gall bladder is contracting against the obstruction.

The most common type of gall stone is composed of cholesterol.

19

Gall bladder removal does not necessarily eliminate symptoms.

In the conventional medical system, the usual recommendation is a cholecystectomy (surgical removal of the gall bladder). Surgery is believed to be a quick and final way of dealing with organic disease such as gall stones. Unfortunately, the true cause of the problem often goes unrecognized and untreated. This is demonstrated by the fact that gall bladder removal does not necessarily eliminate symptoms. The Mayo Clinic has found that 56 percent of patients who have had their gall bladder removed continue to experience many of the same symptoms they had prior to the operation such as indigestion, constipation and intolerance to fat.

Gall bladder removal allows bile to drip 24 hours a day into the digestive tract. This can be very irritating to sections of the bowel. A constant irritation to any tissue can initiate a precancerous condition. Indeed, studies from England, Germany and the US show a doubling of the rate of cancer of the large intestine after 10 or 20 years in such patients. For this reason, cholecystectomies are among the most questioned types of operations. Non-invasive treatments for gall stones are available such as bile acid, contact solvent and shock wave therapy but the recurrence rate for these patients, who may receive little or no dietary counseling, is approximately 50 percent within 10 to 15 years.

Liver/Gall Bladder Flush

Many natural health practitioners recommend a liver/gall bladder flush using lemon juice and olive oil to squeeze the stones out. A typical recipe for a liver/gall bladder flush is:

1 lemon, juiced
2 oranges, juiced
2 tablespoons olive oil
2 tablespoons water
¼" slice fresh, peeled ginger root, minced
Pinch cayenne

Blend above ingredients and drink on an empty stomach in the morning. Garlic pills may also be taken with the concoction followed by a cup of herb tea. Some queasiness may be experienced due to the release of toxins. This usually passes upon drinking the tea. Wait one hour before taking any solid food. Repeat the process each morning for one week. Ordinarily, the stones begin to pass after the third day and can be seen in the stool.

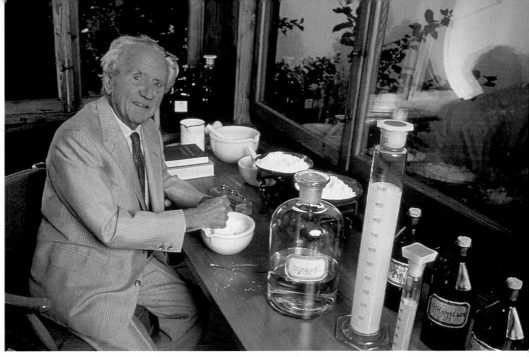

Dr. H.C.A. Vogel, the famous Swiss nature doctor, recommended 8 to 12 ounces (300 to 500 ml) of unrefined oil (such as flax, olive or walnut oils) all at once to stimulate a flood of bile and eliminate small- to medium-sized stones with it. If this quantity of oil is too disagreeable, the same quantity can be taken spaced out over several days (as described in previous box) but with somewhat less effective results. Another alternative is to consume about ¼ cup (60 ml) every 15 minutes or so. After consuming the oil, lie on the right side. For best results, it is important to give the bowels a good clean-out beforehand using an enema or laxative.

Although rare, there is a possibility that a vigorous gall bladder flush could cause large stones to get stuck requiring a quick trip to the hospital for removal. Also, muscle contractility is sometimes a problem in older people and the gall bladder is not able to expel the stones. To minimize the possibility of stones getting stuck, it is advisable to tone up the liver and gall bladder for several weeks prior to a flush using lecithin granules, choloretic herbs and lipotropic supplements. These products help thin the bile and make it less sticky. Like the oil treatment, the herbs stimulate bile flow. Whether a person chooses to do a gall bladder flush or not, these supplements are invaluable in supporting liver/gall bladder function.

Natural health pioneer Dr. Alfred Vogel recommended unrefined oil to eliminate gall stones.

21

Lipotropic supplements consist of choline, inositol, betaine, methionine, and sometimes herbs. Hepatic and choleretic herbs include artichoke, barberry, dandelion, milk thistle seed, boldo, greater celandine and fringe-tree. Homeopathic gall stone medication may also be incorporated. In addition, there are reports of radish juice dissolving gall stones over a six week course. In macrobiotics, daikon, a large, white radish is recommended. For those who have had their gall bladder removed, several ounces of aloe vera juice or gel taken daily will help to soothe irritated bowel tissue.

Hepatic and choleretic herbs, such as artichoke, tone the liver.

Carrot/Daikon Drink

½ cup grated carrot
½ cup grated daikon radish
2 cups water
⅓ sheet nori sea vegetable
½ umeboshi plum
A few drops of shoyu/soy sauce

Combine carrot, daikon and water in a saucepan. Bring to a boil. Add nori and umeboshi plum. Simmer about 3 minutes then add shoyu/soy sauce. Eat and drink the vegetables and broth. Take every day for ten days or every other day for three weeks.

James Breneman, MD, past chairperson of the Food Allergy Committee of the American College of Allergists contends that gall bladder attacks can be completely avoided by eliminating foods to which a person is allergic. In a trial, Dr. Breneman put 51 patients with gall stones and 18 who had their gall bladders removed but still suffered with pain on an elimination diet made up of foods he felt had a minimum allergic potential such beef, rye, soybean, rice and spinach. At the end of one week all patients (100 percent) were relieved of their symptoms. Foods that were ordinarily eaten were added back one at a time to identify ones that provoked an attack. On average, four to five foods had to be excluded. Two foods that patients most commonly reacted to were eggs (93 percent) and pork (64 percent). The list that followed included onions, poultry, milk, coffee, oranges, corn, beans and nuts. Occasionally, medications were to blame for the allergic reaction.

Gall stones, appendicitis, hiatal hernia, hemorrhoids and various diseases of the colon are extremely rare in parts of the world where the population consumes a high-fiber diet. The importance of dietary fiber for these kinds of digestive disorders is now widely recognized and constipation has been linked to gall stones.

Sugar consumption may also pose a risk for gall stone development. Sugar promotes insulin secretion, which increases cholesterol synthesis in the liver—a condition favoring stone formation. Studies report a higher prevalence of gall stones in people with a high sugar diet.

Since gall stones actually represent a liver problem, it is important to minimize dietary stress to this organ. The liver can be harmed by too much saturated fat, a deficiency of vitamins, minerals and essential unsaturated fats, excessive amounts of alcohol, sugar, refined carbohydrates, drugs, chemicals and food additives. Virtually, everything we eat, drink and breathe must be dealt with by the liver. For complete, easy-to-understand information on this topic, read *Liver Cleansing Handbook*, by Rhody Lake (*alive* Natural Health Guides #4, 2000).

Millions of North Americans visit doctors for chronic heartburn each year.

Heartburn

Heartburn is acid indigestion that causes irritation of the esophagus, the tube leading from the mouth to the stomach. Most of us have experienced this sour, burning sensation after over-indulgence with food or drink at one time or another. The stomach lining is usually protected from the effects of its own acid but certain factors cause us to lose this protection. The esophagus, however, is not protected against acid and a back-flow from the stomach causes irritation felt in the chest. Each year, tens of millions of North Americans visit doctors for chronic heartburn, also called gastroesophageal reflux disease.

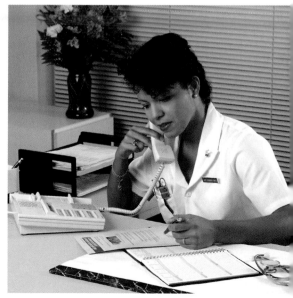

Occasional heartburn does not pose a serious health risk, but if you experience it frequently, two or more times a week, it can be extremely hazardous to your health. Constant irritation of the food pipe can cause ulceration and progress to esophageal cancer, a highly fatal disease now being seen in epidemic numbers, particularly in men 30 to 50 years of age. In the US, it is the fastest growing cancer.

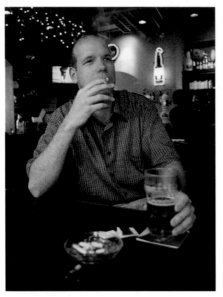

Risk factors for heartburn include obesity, alcohol consumption and tobacco use.

Normally, a muscular valve at the end of the esophagus keeps food and liquids in the stomach and out of the esophagus. Reflux can occur when the valve relaxes for a moment, when it is faulty or injured, or if a person increases pressure on the stomach by straining, bending over or eating too large a meal. Risk factors include certain medicines, age (older than 65), obesity, pregnancy, a high-fat diet and excessive consumption of caffeine, alcohol or tobacco.

Conventional treatment of acid reflux is with nonabsorbable antacids or antisecretory drugs that block production of stomach acid. Treatment of heartburn with such medications is palliative and does not address underlying conditions that cause acid indigestion. Advertisements proclaim there are no good reasons not to take Zantac, but acid-blockers can cause adverse reactions and disrupt ecological balance in the gut.

Reducing or stopping the natural secretion of stomach acid gives cause for concern. Hydrochloric acid (HCl) secretion by the stomach is required for proper assimilation of minerals and protein and serves to protect against micro-organisms by sterilizing the food we've eaten. Stomach acid secretion is also important because it signals the pancreas to secrete its digestive enzymes.

A natural, preventive approach to acid indigestion and reflux incorporates enzymes and often HCl. Rather than shutting down the digestive process with acid-blockers or antacids, enzymes and HCl facilitate digestion.

Most people who suffer from heartburn or acid indigestion think they produce too much acid. However, this is often not the case. Studies show that most people taking antacids are actually deficient in HCl. As we get older, we tend to produce less stomach acid, not more. The same is true for many enzymes and hormones. More than half the population over age 60 have insufficient secretory abilities. According to an article in *The New England Journal of Medicine*, as many as 30 to 40 percent of postmenopausal women have low to no stomach acid secretion unless the stomach is given some type of stimulus. If food is not being digested quickly enough and remains in the stomach too long, fermentation acids develop (the bad acid). Also, we may experience a delayed secretion of our own stomach acid after fermentation has occurred, compounding the problem.

As we age we produce less of the stomach acid that aids the digestive process.

So, how do you spell "relief?" P-r-e-v-e-n-t-i-o-n is the key to eradicating acid indigestion and heartburn. Once you have heartburn, there is little that can be done except to take a drug or wait it out. Bicarbonate of soda (baking soda) or other antacids may provide temporary relief. To prevent heartburn, adhere to the 10 Commandments for Good Digestion (see page 14). Do not lie down after eating a large meal since gravity does not favor a weak esophageal sphincter muscle. To avoid trouble at night, do not eat a large meal within three hours of bedtime. Nighttime is for resting the digestive organs, not working overtime. See a physician if heartburn symptoms persist.

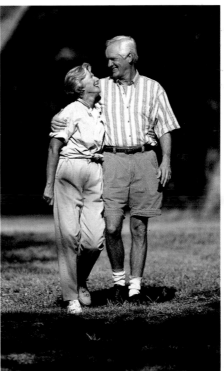

Hemorrhoids

Hemorrhoids are protruding, varicose veins in the anal area. Symptoms include burning, itching, pain and blood in the stool. The most frequent cause is straining during bowel movements, common among people who are constipated or pregnant.

Hemorrhoids could also be representative of liver dysfunction. If the blood becomes congested with fats, more pressure is placed on the blood vessels.

To prevent and treat hemorrhoids, obtain plenty of fiber in the diet or add a daily fiber supplement. A folk remedy for hemorrhoids is placing a peeled and oiled clove of garlic in the rectum as a suppository. In case of a severe condition, fasting may be the quickest way to correct the problem.

To strengthen veins and reduce swelling use Enzymatic Therapy's *Hem-Tone* and/or an herbal remedy such as *Collinsonia/ Horse Chestnut Compound* from Herb Pharm. Other accessory supplements that strengthen connective tissue and blood vessels are pycnogenol or grapeseed extract (100-300 mg/day).

Inflammatory Bowel Disease

Inflammation is a response to irritation causing pain, redness and swelling and eventually destruction of tissue. Inflammatory bowel disease (IBD) is inflammation affecting the small intestine or colon. The two most common types of IBD are Crohn's disease and ulcerative colitis. The diseases are similar but have different characteristics. IBD bears no direct relationship with irritable bowel syndrome (IBS) which is a motility disorder. Most theories suggest that increased permeability of the intestinal mucosa, often called "leaky gut," underlies the disease process. (See "Leaky Gut Syndrome" on page 31.)

As the name implies, ulcerative colitis affects only the colon (large intestine). The inflammation affects the innermost lining of the colon and is most severe in the rectum, extending up the colon in a continuous manner without any skip pattern. Crohn's disease can affect any part of the gastrointestinal tract, including the small intestine. Unlike ulcerative colitis, it is not continuous and there may be areas of normal tissue between diseased patches. Also, Crohn's disease can affect the entire thickness of the bowel wall.

Symptoms of IBD include abdominal pain, cramping and diarrhea which may also be accompanied by bleeding. Often, there are complications and hospitalization is required. Conventional medical treatment for IBD consists of anti-inflammatory and immune-suppressive drugs, steroids and sometimes antibiotics.

Some patients undergo surgery due to massive bleeding.

Diet plays an important role in IBD. The incidence of the disease is growing rapidly in Western countries but is rare in populations where people eat a native diet. There are correlations between IBD and the high-sugar, high-saturated fat and low-fiber diet of North Americans. Food sensitivities also play a significant role and many patients report improvements following an elimination diet.

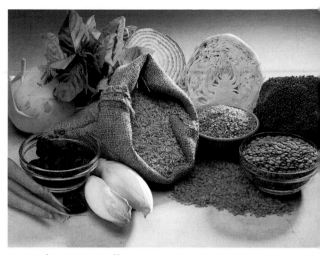

A diet high in fiber plays a positive role in treating and preventing inflammatory bowel disease.

The elimination diet excludes sugars and common allergenic foods for three weeks. A typical elimination diet restricts all foods except vegetables, fruits (no citrus), fish (no shellfish), white rice and rice protein powder. Foods are then added back one at a time to see which ones provoke a response. The foods tested are taken in a pure state and in a generous amount. Allergic reactions to watch for are hives, digestive discomfort, "brain fog" and an increased pulse rate. At least three hours should pass before testing another food. The most commonly allergic foods are (in descending order): milk, wheat, yeast, soy, coffee, tea, chocolate, shellfish, citrus, corn, egg and beef. Do not attempt a food allergy self-test if you have a history of severe allergic reactions, asthma or epilepsy.

There is no one diet that helps all people with IBD. The Specific Carbohydrate Diet outlined in Elaine Gottschall's book *Breaking the Vicious Cycle* works especially well for people with Crohn's disease. While the diet/disease connection has not been proved in IBD, there is strong evidence that modifying the diet can be highly beneficial to patients. There is no doubt that one's food choices influence body chemistry and can alter it to a more favorable state. For example, foods high in arachidonic acid, such as meat, milk and eggs, tend to heighten inflammation whereas fish, fruit and flax oil (omega-3 fatty acids) inhibit inflammation.

A study reported in the *New England Journal of Medicine* demonstrated that a fish oil supplement reduced relapse rates of

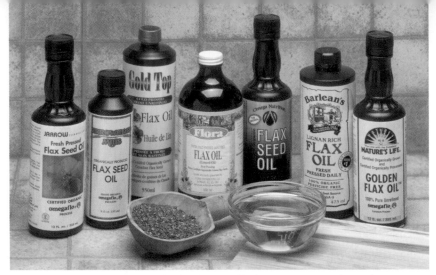

The omega-3 fatty acids in flax oil inhibit the inflammation associated with inflammatory bowel disease.

Crohn's disease. The study enrolled 78 patients whose disease was in remission. Half of the patients were randomly assigned to take nine 500 mg fish oil capsules daily providing a daily total of 2.7 grams of omega-3 fatty acids. The others took nine placebo capsules. After one year of treatment, 74 percent of those taking the placebo had relapsed into acute illness compared to 41 percent of those taking fish oil. Laboratory indicators of inflammation also decreased in the fish oil group. The publication of this research in a prestigious medical journal is encouraging because it shows increasing acceptance of natural treatments by the medical establishment.

Often, bacterial infections are involved, strongly suggesting a need for probiotic products such as Jarrow Formulas Jarrodophilus. One species of friendly bacteria that is especially helpful in controlling diarrhea is *Saccharomyces boulardi*.

Another feature of IBD is poor nutrient absorption. The nutrients required to heal are often malabsorbed, contributing to a downward cycle in the disease. Studies have shown an increased need for antioxidant nutrients vitamins A and E, selenium, zinc, glutathione and superoxide dismutase. Prolonged bleeding can also cause anemia and a need for blood builders iron, copper and B_{12}.

Two nutrients that are partners in repairing intestinal tissue are folic acid and glutamine. Clinical studies have used large doses of folic acid (as high as 15 mg per day). For routine supplementing, 1 mg. (1,000 micrograms) of folic acid is a reasonable dose. The drug Azulfidine, often prescribed for IBD, causes a 30 percent loss of folic acid. Folic acid deficiency can create a high level of homocysteine, a toxic substance in the blood that is a risk factor for cardiovascular disease. In women, a deficiency of folic acid during pregnancy increases the risk of neural tube birth defects.

Glutamine may also improve intestinal health. It serves as a source of fuel for cells lining the stomach and intestines. Without it, these cells waste away.

Other important products for IBD that are soothing and healing are aloe vera juice, chlorophyll and demulcent herbs such as slippery elm, mullein and marshmallow. Aloe vera juice can be obtained conveniently in combination with herbs in a product called *Stomach Formula* by Naturade.

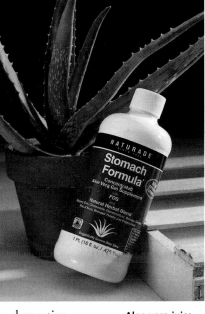

Irritable Bowel Syndrome

Irritable bowel syndrome (IBS) is a common disorder of bowel function for which there is no reliable medical treatment. Symptoms associated with IBS are chronic or recurrent abdominal pain, spasms, bloating, gas and disturbed defecation (constipation/diarrhea). IBS is also known as nervous indigestion and spastic colon and is the most common gastrointestinal disorder seen in general practice.

IBS may be caused by physiological, psychological and/or dietary factors. Other disorders that mimic IBS should be ruled out by a physician. These include inflammatory bowel disease, intestinal candidiasis, celiac disease, diabetes, pancreatic insufficiency, thyroid and adrenal disturbances, diverticulitis, parasite infection and lactose intolerance.

Often, dietary factors such as excessive tea, coffee and/or sugar consumption are to blame. Food sensitivities are found in the majority of IBS patients. The most common trigger foods are wheat, corn, dairy products, coffee, tea, citrus and chocolate. Also, a high percentage of people are unable to breakdown two-sugar molecules, called disaccharides, including mannitol,

Aloe vera juice is both soothing and healing for inflammatory bowel disease.

sucrose, sorbitol and fructose. Like other bowel disorders, a natural approach to IBS involves increasing dietary fiber, eliminating allergic/intolerant foods, herbal therapy, multivitamins and minerals, probiotics and stress management/behavioral modification.

An enteric-coated peppermint oil capsule has been used in treating IBS in Europe. In the US and Canada, it is available from Enzymatic Therapy, Green Bay, Wisconsin. Peppermint oil inhibits gastrointestinal cramping and relieves gas. The usual dose is two to three capsules taken between meals.

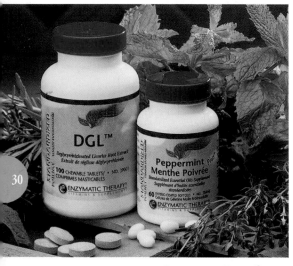

Peppermint and licorice treat symptoms of irritable bowel syndrome.

Results of a randomized, controlled trial using a standard Chinese herbal formula in IBS patients were published in *The Journal of the American Medical Association*. After 16 weeks, patients receiving the formula improved by 59 percent according to gastroenterologists in contrast to patients in a placebo group who improved 19 percent. Patients reported that treatment significantly reduced the degree of interference in their lives and activities caused by IBS symptoms. One company that offers the formula is Samra, called *Calm Colon*.

Lactose Intolerance

If you experience bloating, gas, cramps or diarrhea after consuming milk, cheese, yogurt or ice cream, you may be one of an estimated 60 million North Americans who is lactose intolerant. Lactose intolerance is an inability to digest lactose (milk sugar) due to insufficient amounts of the enzyme lact*ase*.

Many people who are lactose intolerant cannot resist an occasional ice cream cone or slice of pizza. In these cases, supplementing with lactase enzyme supplements make dairy foods more digestible. Tablets may be swallowed or chewed just prior to eating a dairy food. Milk may be pretreated with drops. Lactose-reduced milk is also available. Manufacturers add enough lactase enzyme to digest 70 percent of the lactose in the milk.

Some dairy products, such as kefir, quark and natural, mild

cheeses are more easily digested, even by those who are lactose intolerant.

If you have trouble digesting food at times, these foods may contain lactose and you may be lactose intolerant. A simple test will help you to determine if you lack lactase or your indigestion is due to other factors.

Are You Lactose Intolerant?

Day One
1. Do not eat anything after 10 pm (or 3 to 4 hours before retiring) on the evening prior to the test.
2. Eat your normal breakfast and include a large, 12-ounce glass of whole, skim or low-fat milk.
3. Over the next six hours, keep track of any discomforts if they occur and how severe they are.

Day Two
1. Do not eat anything after 10 pm (3 to 4 hours before retiring) on the evening prior to the test.
2. Swallow or chew the recommended dose of a lactase enzyme supplement five minutes prior to your morning meal.
3. Eat an identical breakfast to what you had on Day One, again including a 12-ounce glass of milk.
   If you are lactose intolerant, you will probably notice less, or even none, of the discomforts you experienced on Day One. If you still experienced some discomfort, you may need to increase the dosage of lactase enzyme you take. If the discomfort continues or you experience symptoms that appear unrelated to lactose intolerance, see your doctor. You might also determine if you are lactose-intolerant by avoiding all dairy foods, and products that contain dairy foods for at least two weeks and observing how you feel.

Leaky Gut Syndrome

Increased intestinal permeability, also called "leaky gut," is a new concept in digestive health believed to contribute to food sensitivities and intestinal diseases as well as many systemic conditions such as fatigue, headaches, eczema and arthritis. It is a condition in which the intestinal lining becomes damaged and loses its ability to act properly as a filter. The increased gut permeability permits large, foreign molecules (bacteria, toxic substances, undigested food) to cross into the systemic circulation and cause allergic reactions. The immune system then becomes "confused" and attacks the body's own cells. A healthy intestinal lining allows only properly digested fats, proteins and starches to pass through. In addition, a leaky gut places an extra burden on the liver to filter inflammatory irritants.

All digestive and systemic conditions can be approached from the concept of improving the integrity of the mucosal barrier. There is no single cause of leaky gut syndrome but the main contributors are chronic stress, dysbiosis (imbalance of intestinal flora), overuse of alcoholic beverages, poor diet, parasites and yeasts, birth control pills and prolonged use of nonsteroidal anti-inflammatory drugs (NSAIDs). Supportive nutrients and supplements include enzymes, probiotics, herbal remedies, antioxidants, multiple vitamins and minerals, gamma oryzanol and glutamine.

Ulcers

Ulcers are lesions in the stomach or upper intestine (duodenum) causing pain, vomiting or bleeding. The open sores are due to the burning effects of stomach acid on an unprotected stomach lining. The stomach wall is usually protected from the effects of its own acid by a mucus barrier but certain factors, such as smoking, stress, and excessive consumption of alcohol, caffeine, salt and aspirin cause this protection to be lost.

For a long time, ulcers were believed to be caused by excessive stomach acid. Today, researchers point the finger at a bacteria called *H. pylori*. This bacteria has been identified in 79 to 90 percent of people with ulcers. When it takes hold, the mucus layer of the stomach is digested and acid comes into contact with the unprotected lining. Interestingly, bacteria tend to thrive in a stomach that lacks stomach acid. Stomach acid secretion is a natural function and the first line of defense against bacteria.

Treatment for ulcers is the same for uncomplicated heartburn, provided that pain is not severe and there is no bleeding. Although acid-blockers Zantac and Tagamet are the most commonly-prescribed medications, the latest approach is to focus on killing *H. pylori* with antibiotics. Despite treatment with drugs, a significant number of people have a relapse of their ulcer within six months.

The sensible approach to ulcers seems to be taking measures to kill *H. pylori* while protecting and restoring the stomach lining. Because ulcers have been experienced throughout history, people have searched and found effective natural remedies. While most physicians are not familiar with such therapies, practitioners of natural medicine obtain good results employing DGL (a form of licorice), grapefruit seed extract, goldenseal (natural antibiotics), slippery elm, aloe vera, chlorophyll, activated charcoal, and mycelized vitamin A (a concentrated, highly-absorbable form of the vitamin). Also, cabbage juice has been a long-standing folk remedy for ulcers ($^1/_2$ cup, three times a day before meals). Work with your physician on tailoring an integrative treatment. If vomiting of black "coffee-ground" material or bright red blood is experienced, call the doctor immediately. Black stools have the same significance (if not taking iron supplements or Pepto Bismol, which also darken the stool).

Cabbage juice is a natural remedy for ulcers.

Natural Remedies for Digestive Support . . . . .

Aloe Vera
Many people are familiar with the soothing and healing properties of aloe vera for external use such as sunburn and other skin conditions. In the kitchen, a quick application of aloe gel to a burn can prevent blistering. Not surprisingly, aloe vera juice confers the same anti-inflammatory properties internally to ulcers and can reduce bleeding time.

Apple Cider Vinegar
Apples are a rich, natural source of potassium and other essential minerals. When whole apples are used to make apple cider vinegar, all of the minerals are retained. The only change is that the sugars of the fruit are rendered into acid. In the digestive tract, acid discourages the growth of bacteria. A couple of teaspoons of apple cider vinegar in water at mealtime can prevent food poisoning. For a case of food poisoning, sips are taken every five minutes until improved, then the intervals between taking the remedy are lengthened. This treatment is safe for children as young as three years. As a remedy and health tonic, the most suitable apple cider vinegar is raw and unfiltered such as that offered by Sterling or Bragg.

The acids in apple cider vinegar also facilitate absorption of the minerals. The acids are metabolized for energy leaving behind the alkalizing minerals. Thus, apple cider vinegar has a beneficial effect on the acid/alkaline balance of the body. This may account for its usefulness in so many conditions and its reputation as a versatile folk remedy.

Betaine HCl

If symptoms in Section One of the Digestive Symptom Survey indicate hypochlorhidria (low stomach acid), a betaine hydrochloride supplement may be of benefit. People who are deficient in stomach acid often complain they feel bloated in the stomach or the food feels like rocks and is not being digested. Sometimes there is burping or hiccups.

As we get older, we tend to produce less stomach acid and thus are often at greater risk for stomach distress, bacterial infections and decreased nutrient assimilation.

Determining whether or not you might benefit from supplemental HCl is a simple matter of taking the pills at meal time to see if it prevents your symptoms. Take one 10-grain (650 mg) capsule or tablet of betaine with the same size, similar composition meal each day, gradually increasing the number of pills daily to determine the amount that eliminates your symptoms. Usually, one or two pills or as many as six is sufficient to improve symptoms of low stomach acid. If betaine causes burning, you probably have too much acid and can neutralize it by taking baking soda or eating a bit more. Betaine and glutamic acid supplements are contraindicated in the presence of peptic or duodenal ulcer.

Chlorophyll

Chlorophyll is the green pigment found in plants. Called "the blood of plants," it is chemically very similar to our own blood. Its molecular structure closely resembles hemin, the pigment that combines with protein to form hemoglobin. Rather than containing iron at the cell center, as found in human blood, chlorophyll contains magnesium. Chlorophyll helps the body to obtain more oxygen and acts as a "magnet" in drawing out toxins from the body. For this reason, it is called "the internal deodorant."

Chlorophyll has a long history as a therapeutic agent for damaged or injured tissues. Its effect is one that is cleansing, soothing and healing. Chlorophyll is highly recommended for ulcers, gastritis, colitis, hemorrhoids, bad breath, dental extractions and oral hygiene. In acute conditions, take one to two tablespoons liquid chlorophyll in water every two hours. Chlorophyll may also be applied to external hemorrhoids or used in enemas.

Alfalfa is the most common source of commercial chlorophyll but other rich sources are green barley, wheatgrass, and freshwater algae such as spirulina and chlorella. Green food supplements are especially valuable during a fast or detoxification program, or whenever we don't consume our quota for green, leafy vegetables.

Enzymes

Enzymes are often referred to as "the key to life and health," "the spark of life" and "the missing link in nutrition." Such phrases are not exaggerations because, without enzymes, life would not be possible. No plant, animal or human could exist without them.

Enzymes are composed of proteins and found in all cells of plants, animals and the human body. Scientists describe enzymes as catalysts that initiate chemical reactions or speed processes. These processes can be seen throughout nature. For example, enzymes are at work when fruit ripens or milk is turned into cheese and yogurt. In the body, millions of enzymes are involved in all anabolic (building) and catabolic (breaking down) processes we call metabolism.

All foods must be digested by enzymes, therefore supplementation is sometimes necessary.

Although our bodies make most of the enzymes we need, many enzymes are available in foods. Fresh, raw fruits and vegetables and their juices are good sources with sprouts having the highest enzyme content. Also, when grains, seeds or nuts are sprouted (germinated), the enzyme levels increase up to five or six times. It makes good sense to eat these enzyme-rich foods in order to avoid overworking the body's enzyme

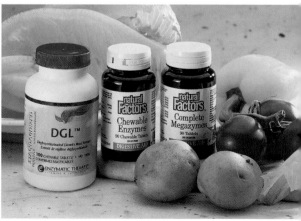

Poor digestion can weaken the body's ability to fight disease.

capacity. The typical Western diet of cooked, highly processed, enzyme-depleted foods are huge contributors to poor health and disease.

The human digestive tract has first priority on enzyme production. After all, food must be digested by enzymes to extract all nutrients necessary to fuel the body. Poor digestion can ultimately weaken the body's ability to fight disease and can result in an overtaxed system. Symptoms such as gas and discomfort after meals are an indication of incomplete digestion and that the body's digestive capacity has been exceeded. Following the 10 Commandments for Good Digestion (see page 14) will go a long way in helping this process but often one benefits from a digestive enzyme supplement. Your score on the Digestive Symptom Survey will help determine which digestive supplement is best suited for you, whether it is pancreatin, food enzymes or betaine.

If you have symptoms in several categories, a comprehensive, multiple digestive enzyme supplement is a good choice. These products contain pancreatic enzymes, betaine hydrochloride or glutamic acid and bile. Examples of such products are Nature's Plus *Ultra Zyme*, Country Life's *MaxiZyme* and Enzymatic Therapy's *Pro-Gest Ade*. Take these products during the meal or after eating (up to an hour after a large meal) to help prevent digestive disturbances and reduce hypersensitive food reactions. Once you have indigestion, it is too late to take the product. If symptoms in Section One of the Digestive Symptom Survey indicate hypochlorhidria (low stomach acid), extra betaine HCl may be necessary (See "Betaine HCl" on page 34).

Even without digestive symptoms, you may wish to take a plant-derived food enzyme supplement for routine use since most people do not consume an optimal amount of enzyme-rich foods. Such products are Source Naturals *Essential Enzymes* or Rainbow Light's *All Zyme*. Take these products just before or at the beginning of a meal.

Fiber

Fiber has been called "the essential non-digestible" because it is not digested and absorbed yet necessary for a healthy gastrointestinal tract. Fiber exercises the colon by stimulating peristalsis, the wave-like, muscular contractions of the intestine. Fiber works like a broom for the intestine, sweeping it clean. Fiber also helps to hold moisture in the colon and loosen and soften debris that may become trapped. Yet another benefit is its ability to act like a sponge, absorbing fats and sugars and slowing their entry into the bloodstream. Fiber also transports cholesterol out of the body. The best sources of fiber are unrefined plant foods: fruits, vegetables, beans and particularly whole grains. Peeling fruits and vegetables removes much of the fiber.

Appendicitis, hiatal hernia, hemorrhoids, gall stones and various diseases of the colon are extremely rare in parts of the world where people consume a high-fiber diet (40 to 60 grams). Recommendations are 20 to 35 grams of fiber per day but the average intake in modern, affluent diets is only about 10 grams. Fiber is not just important for your digestive tract. Studies show an inverse relation of fiber to heart disease and some types of cancer.

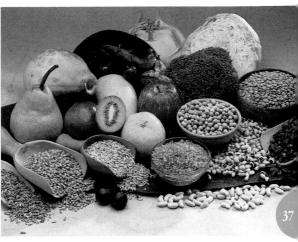

The best sources of fiber include fruit, vegetables, beans and whole grains.

When a person is unwilling or unable to make the necessary changes in the diet, a fiber supplement becomes necessary. Start by adding one teaspoon of oat bran, wheat bran or psyllium to your breakfast or stir it into juice or water. Once you know you tolerate it, begin increasing the amount daily until bowel movements are effortless and odorless. Drink plenty of water throughout the day for best results. Sometimes fiber supplements, or switching to a high-fiber diet, can cause temporary gas due to a change in the bacterial population of the bowel. If a fiber supplement causes digestive upset or constipation, reduce the dosage to what is tolerated. Often, this is an indication of a need for digestive enzymes.

Gamma-Oryzanol

Gamma-o is a component of rice bran, corn and barley oils and is a mixture of sterols (hormone-like substances) and ferulic acid. Research suggests that it increases testosterone levels, the release of endorphins ("feel good hormones") and the growth of lean muscle tissue. Clinical experience indicates that gamma-o is healing to the intestinal lining and may be beneficial in celiac disease, diverticular disease, IBD, IBS, gastritis and ulcer. Much of the human research with gamma-o used 300 mg per day. For a trial, take 100 mg three times per day for several weeks.

Ginger

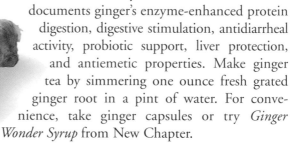

Ginger is of great benefit to the stomach and intestines and can be taken for indigestion, nausea and cramps. Unlike any drug, ginger is both anti-inflammatory and antiulcer. Research documents ginger's enzyme-enhanced protein digestion, digestive stimulation, antidiarrheal activity, probiotic support, liver protection, and antiemetic properties. Make ginger tea by simmering one ounce fresh grated ginger root in a pint of water. For convenience, take ginger capsules or try *Ginger Wonder Syrup* from New Chapter.

Glutamine

Glutamine is an amino acid brain fuel, growth hormone releaser and gut healer. It is the preferred food of the cells of the small intestine. Although few people are deficient in glutamine, supplemental doses are known to be helpful for peptic ulcer and ulcerative colitis. Suggested dosages usually range from 1 gram to 20 grams. However, even small doses of 500 mg three times per day are known to prevent colitis in cancer patients receiving abdominal radiation. Start with one teaspoon powder (5 grams) in water twice a day between meals on an empty stomach for a four-week trial. Adjust dose as required.

Licorice

Licorice is a proven remedy for stomach and intestinal ulcers. It also supports liver and adrenal gland function and helps counteract stress. However, large doses can exacerbate hypertension. Deglycyrrhizinated licorice (DGL) is without the possible side effect because the component that can increase blood pressure has been removed. DGL can make it possible to reduce or eliminate antacids. In clinical studies, DGL has been shown to be as effective or more effective than Tagamet, Zantac or antacids for both short term treatment and maintenance therapy of gastric ulcer. DGL does not block acid production but instead protects and heals the stomach lining. DGL lozenges are available from Enzymatic Therapy. Chew two tablets twenty minutes before meals. Mixing the licorice with saliva seems to be important in its effectiveness. Continue treatment for eight to sixteen weeks.

Peppermint

Peppermint tea is used to expel gas and griping in the bowel. In Europe, an enteric-coated peppermint oil capsule has been used to prevent spasms in irritable bowel syndrome. Instead of being released in the stomach, the pill is designed to dissolve in the small intestine and colon where the oil acts as a bowel relaxant. The capsules are available in health stores from Enzymatic Therapy. The standard dose is two to three capsules taken between meals. Occasionally, unabsorbed menthol from the peppermint causes a burning sensation in the rectum during defecation. If this should occur, reduce the dose.

Probiotics

When an infection threatens your body, a doctor's weapon of choice is usually an antibiotic. Antibiotics (meaning "against life") swiftly and efficiently kill or inhibit the growth of disease-causing bacteria in the same way a lethal bomb destroys the enemy and their arsenal—all at once. However, also like bombs, many of these drugs aren't selective enough about what they demolish. Often, antibiotics not only wipe out the bacteria that cause infections, but also the body's own good bacteria, which help to maintain a sanitary, ecologically balanced internal environment.

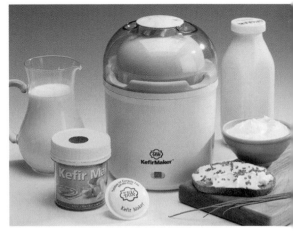

Kefir and other fermented foods promote friendly bacteria in the gut.

In order to restore these friendly micro-organisms to the intestinal tract and help prevent further infections, natural healthcare practitioners often recommend using the opposite of antibiotics—appropriately named *probiotics*. Beyond replacing the good bacteria that antibiotics remove, these natural supplements contain live bacteria that compete with disease-causing organisms and can have far-reaching benefits for immunity and overall health.

Two groups or genuses of bacteria are commonly used in probiotic supplements: *Lactobacilli* and *Bifidobacteria*. The *Lactobacilli* genus, made up of bacteria that produce lactic acid when they ferment carbohydrates, includes two common species, *L. acidophilus* and *L. bulgaricus*, both of which are often found in yogurt. More than 30 different *Bifidobacteria* have been isolated, but among the species most often found in humans are *B. longum*, *B. breve* and *B. bifidum*. Each species tends to colonize its own region of the intestines. *Bifidobacteria* are most numerous in the large intestine, while *Lactobacilli* prevail in the small intestine.

Supplementation with Healthful Bacteria

Reimplantation of healthful bacteria after antibiotic treatment is essential, but most people also can benefit from the routine use of a probiotic. Studies show that maintaining a healthy balance of *Lactobacilli* and *Bifidobacteria* can:

1. help treat vaginitis, urethritis, cystitis, *C. albicans*, staph and gonorrhea
2. reduce cholesterol
3. produce natural antibiotics (called bacteriocins) that control disease-causing organisms
4. alleviate constipation and diarrhea, especially if caused by antibiotic use
5. prevent and reduce the severity of *tourista* (dysentery) when traveling to other countries
6. help the body digest lactose (milk sugar)
7. improve absorption of food and minerals
8. possibly reduce risk of ulcers
9. possibly reduce the risk of colorectal cancer

A diet high in refined carbohydrates and low in fiber reduces the number of friendly bacteria in the gut (intestines and stomach), upsetting the balance of the body's intestinal ecosystem. Other factors contribute to a deficiency of probiotic bacteria such as alcohol, radiation, chlorinated water, birth control pills, cortisone, stress and aging. However, the greatest threat to healthy flora is the indiscriminate use of antibiotics. Some antibiotics do not differentiate between good and bad bacteria and may kill all the good bacteria, but leave behind dangerous coliform bacteria, such as *E. coli*. This compromises the digestive tract's defenses and, although the consequences may not be immediately obvious, can leave the body more susceptible to further problems such as staph and yeast infections (candidiasis).

Probiotic supplements can be taken daily; no friendly bacteria remain in the gut permanently, so regular supplementation will maintain a high level. An excess of good bacteria won't harm you, but taking too much could cause loose bowels.

Yogurt, kefir and other fermented foods, such as sauerkraut and dill pickles, can provide friendly bacteria, too. However, don't count on store-bought yogurt or commercial foods to contain live bacteria in significant numbers. Some supermarket varieties have been sterilized to extend shelf life, which kills their beneficial bacteria. A quality yogurt should state that it contains live cultures. Stay away from yogurt that is mixed with fruit or thickened with gelatin. Look for "natural" yogurt. The only way to be sure you're getting the right bacteria in the right numbers is to use probiotic supplements. With regular supplementation, your friendly bacteria will flourish–and so will you.

Slippery Elm Bark

Slippery elm is a nutritious demulcent and antinausea food. It is soothing to irritated tissues of the stomach and intestines and is a folk remedy in European and Native American cultures. Mix the powder with a little water and take as a tea. You can also purchase slippery elm lozenges.

Good Eating . . . .

I hope I've helped you understand that digestion is a key issue in any type of health problem and one the most important factors influencing your total well-being. In fact, digestion is the key to vibrant health.

If you can resolve difficulties with digestion and elimination, you will achieve a great advantage in overcoming other health problems, whether minor or severe. When a person maintains efficient digestion, a strong body chemistry is the result and all other systems begin to benefit. Digestion is a critical facet of nutrition. So don't just pay attention to what you eat, but how you are digesting it as well. Get to know your digestive system and the symptoms and clues it gives you. You will feel better for it. Good eating!

Digestion is one of the most important factors influencing your total well-being.

41

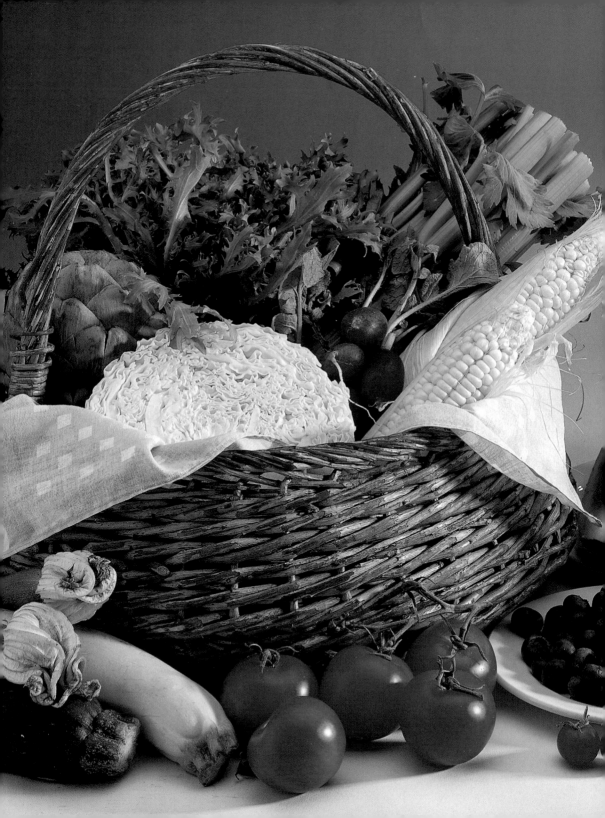

Digestion is a critical facet of nutrition.

Flax-Yogurt-Fruit Bowl

You can prepare this nourishing breakfast in a hurry and with any fresh fruit on hand. Yogurt contains beneficial bacteria for the intestines and gut, and the flax is a delicious source of fiber, protein and omega-3 fatty acids.

1 cup (250 ml) **natural plain yogurt or kefir**

1 tbsp flax seeds, freshly ground

½ cup (125 ml) **fresh sliced fruit of your choice, such as bananas, apple or in-season berries**

Combine the ingredients in a bowl and enjoy.

Serves 2

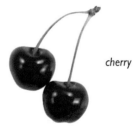

cherry

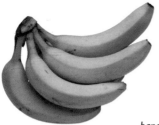

banana

To freshly grind your flax seeds, use a coffee grinder and pulse the seeds for 2 seconds–no longer. This will turn the seeds into a coarse powder.

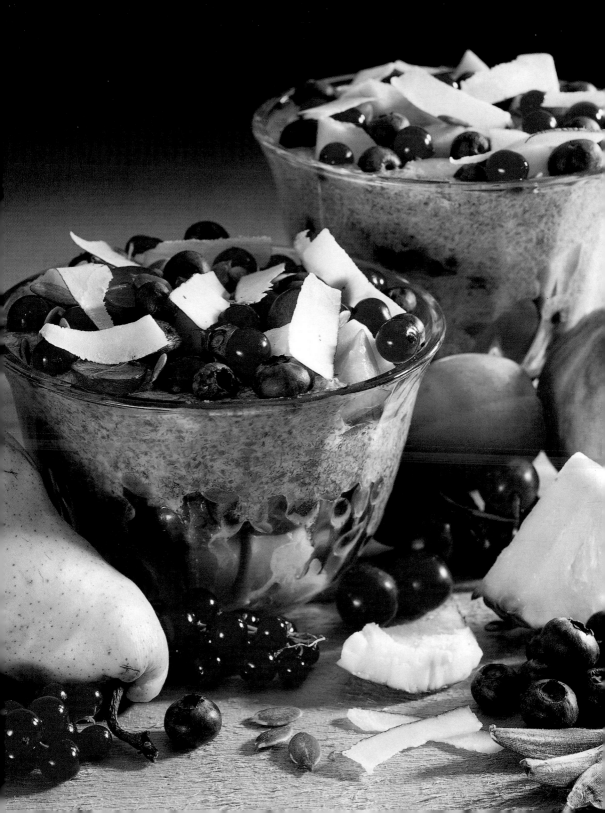

Watermelon Juice with Blueberry-Kefir "Hero's Breakfast"

Watermelon is quickly and easily digested, and has excellent alkalizing and diuretic properties. Drink this juice by itself when you get up in the morning and it will ease the complex burdens of digestion, assimilation and elimination, enabling you to efficiently cleanse, heal and build.

4 cups (1 l) **watermelon, freshly juiced**

2 cups (500 ml) **blueberries**

1 cup (250 ml) **kefir**

2 tbsp pumpkin seeds

Combine blueberries and kefir in bowls and sprinkle with pumpkin seeds. Serve immediately with the watermelon juice.

Serves 2

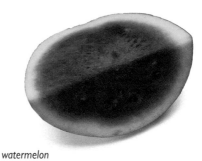

watermelon

Kefir is a living food made of fermented milk that is very easy to digest. It is easy to make your own homemade kefir. Look for kefir culture in health food stores.

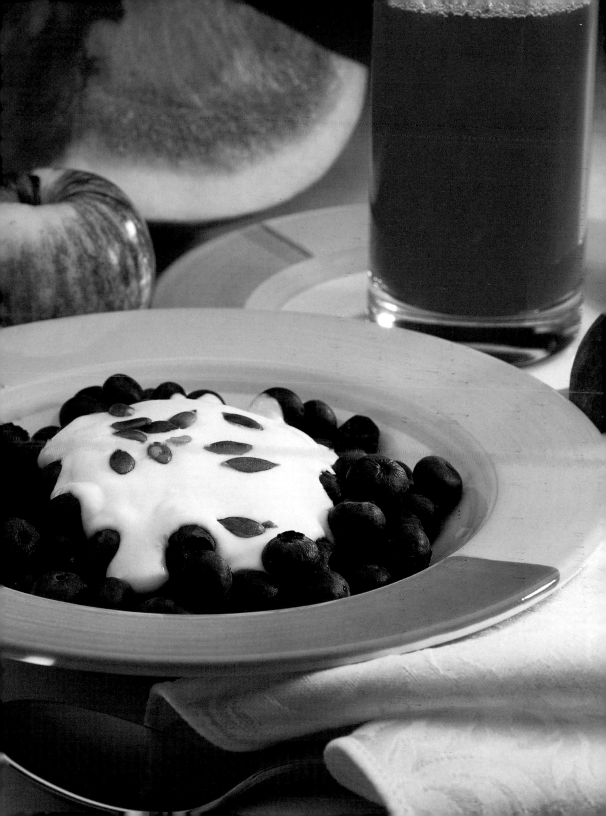

Daikon Soup with Rice Noodles

A large white radish from Asia, daikon is known to aid digestion with its diuretic action and enzymes, and it is especially recommended in the treatment of gall stones. Look for firm roots that are heavy for their size.

2 cups (500 ml) **rice noodles**

1 cup (250 ml) **daikon, julienned**

1 cup (250 ml) **carrot, julienned**

1 cup (250 ml) **cucumber, julienned**

2 cups (500 ml) **Macrobiotic Broth** (recipe below)

1 tbsp rice wine vinegar

1 tbsp extra-virgin olive oil (or flax or sesame seed oil)

1 tsp wheat-free tamari or soy sauce

2 tbsp green onion, chopped

Place rice noodles, daikon, carrot and cucumber in a large bowl and pour salted boiling water over top. Soak for 7 to 10 minutes then drain and set aside.

In the meantime, heat broth in a pot then stir in rice noodles, vegetables, vinegar, oil and tamari. Sprinkle with green onion and serve.

Serves 2

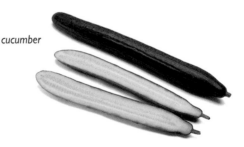

cucumber

Macrobiotic Broth

Eat and drink the vegetables and broth to treat gall stones. Take every day for ten days or every other day for three weeks. You can find these ingredients in a health food store that carries macrobiotic staples.

In a saucepan, combine carrot, daikon and water; bring to a boil. Add nori and plum. Simmer for about 3 minutes than add tamari.

½ cup (125 ml) carrots, grated
½ cup (125 ml) daikon, grated
2 cups (500 ml) water
⅓ sheet nori sea vegetable
½ umeboshi plum
Dash wheat-free tamari or soy sauce

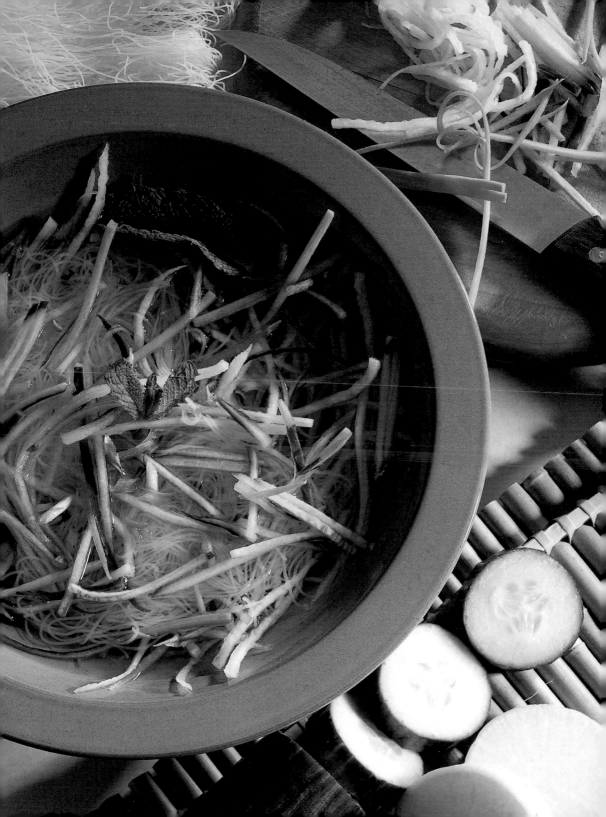

Chayote Salad with Fruit

Chayote, also known as vegetable pear, is similar to summer squash. The flavors in this salad complement each other very well—tangy, sweet, fruity, juicy, leaving a refreshing taste and feel that will stay with you for a long time.

2 cups (500 ml) **curly endive** (frisée lettuce)

1 ripe Granny Smith apple, thinly sliced

1 large pink grapefruit, peeled and segmented

1 large chayote, peeled and thinly sliced

1 red bell pepper, julienned, for garnish

Dressing:

1 tbsp water

1 tbsp honey

¼ cup (60 ml) **apple cider**

1 small shallot, minced

¼ cup (60 ml) **cold-pressed walnut or pistachio oil**

To make the dressing, warm water with honey on low heat, add apple cider and shallot and warm for 3 to 4 minutes. Remove from heat, add oil and mix thoroughly. You can use a hand mixer to emulsify.

Place endive, apple, grapefruit and chayote onto plates then drizzle dressing over top and garnish with red pepper. I also recommend sprinkling this salad with some chopped dry lavender.

Serves 2

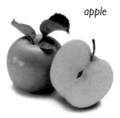

apple

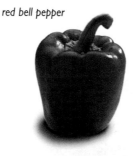

red bell pepper

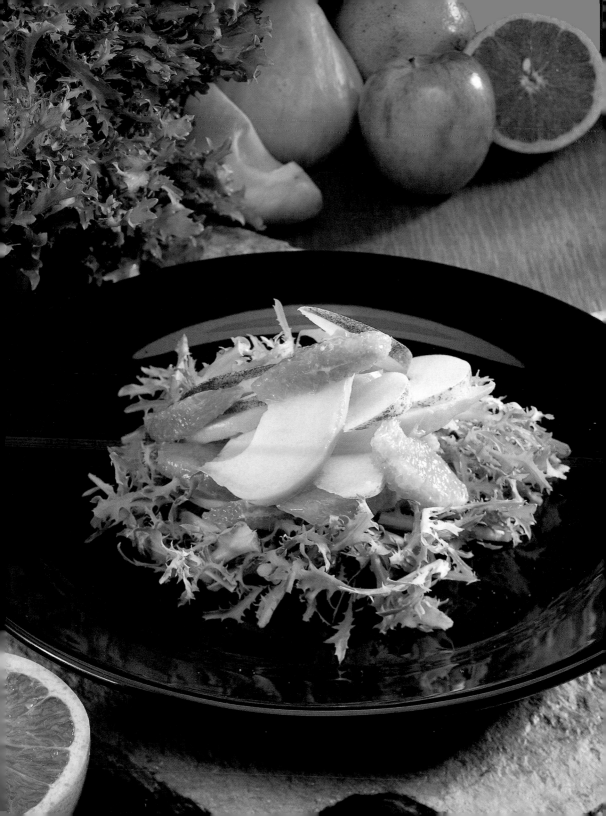

Potato Salad with Kefir

This variation of an old favorite is quick, easy and nutritious. In addition to providing carbohydrates and protein, the potato has significant quantities of minerals found just underneath the skin.

2 lbs (1 kg) **red nugget potatoes, cut in wedges**

1 cup (250 ml) **natural organic yogurt or kefir**

¼ cup (60 ml) **green onion, chopped**

¼ cup (60 ml) **white onion, chopped**

1 clove garlic, minced

1 tbsp flax seed oil

1 tbsp fresh parsley, chopped

1 tbsp fresh chives, chopped

Herbamare, to taste

Cook potato in a pot of salted water for 8 to 10 minutes. Drain and immediately rinse with cold water. Set aside.

In a bowl, thoroughly combine remaining ingredients. Add potato and toss well. Leave at room temperature for at least ½ hour before serving in order for the flavors to fully incorporate.

Serves 4

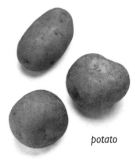

potato

Herbamare is a seasoning made with sea salt and 14 organic herbs. The special steeping process used to make this natural product allows the full herb and vegetable flavor to become concentrated in the salt crystal–preserving essential vitamins and minerals and providing ultimate zest.

Using natural yogurt or kefir to speed up digestion is an ancient remedy. A mixture of yogurt and cooked rice is a gentle and tasty way to remedy constipation. After thousands of years, this concoction still works!

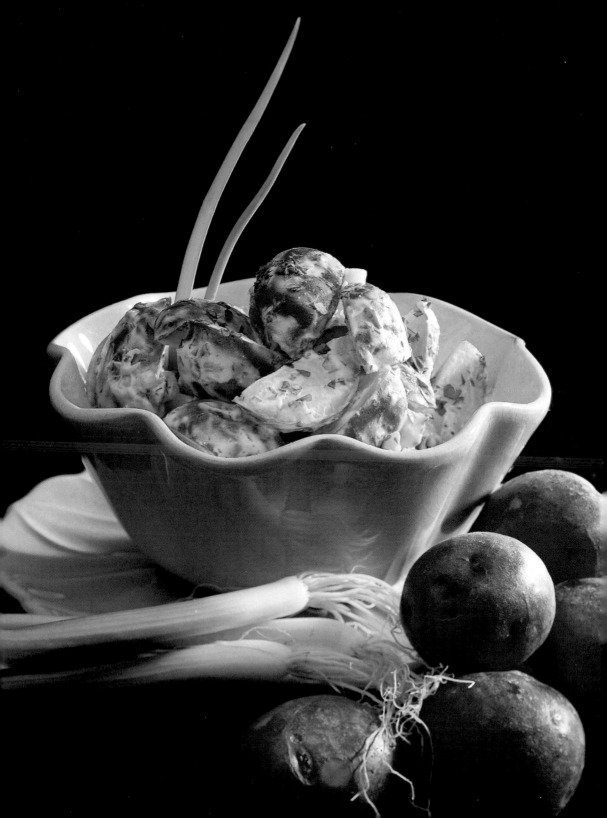

Steamed Vegetables with Carrot-Daikon Salad

Raw daikon commonly accompanies many Japanese and macrobiotic dishes. This simple salad will stimulate your digestive juices.

Vegetable/Noodle Dish:

10 stems green onion

2 cups (500 ml) **rice noodles**

2 cups (500 ml) **broccoli florets**

6 baby carrots

4 pieces baby bok choy

4 pattypans (scallop squash)

2 cups (500 ml) **bean sprouts**

Black and white sesame seeds, for garnish

Salad:

1 medium daikon, julienned

1 carrot, julienned

1 medium chayote, peeled and julienned

Dressing:

4 tbsp rice wine vinegar

2 tbsp toasted sesame seed oil

Sea salt and freshly ground pepper, to taste

Dash fresh lemon or lime juice (optional)

Cut the bulbs off the green onions, removing the roots. Chop 2 tablespoons of the stems and set aside, reserving the remaining stems. Bring a pot of water to a boil with a dash of tamari and blanch the onion bulbs for 3 to 4 minutes. Drain and immediately rinse with cold water. Set aside.

Place rice noodles in a large bowl and pour salted boiling water over top. Soak for 7 to 10 minutes then drain and set aside.

In the meantime, steam broccoli, carrots, bok choy, squash and bean sprouts for 5 minutes.

To make the salad, combine dressing ingredients in a bowl then add daikon, carrot and chayote and toss well.

Arrange rice noodles, onions and steamed vegetables on plates. Sprinkle with sesame seeds and serve with the salad.

Serves 2

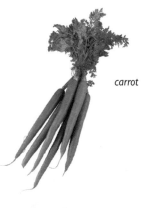

carrot

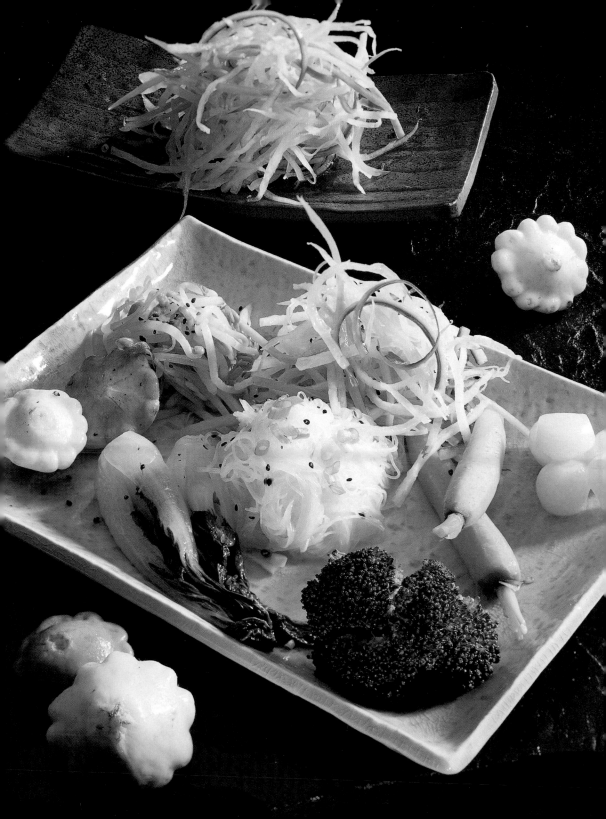

Quinoa-Vegetable Risotto with Braised Halibut

The ginger in the tomato salsa stimulates digestion, protects the liver and is both anti-inflammatory and antiulcer. The zesty salsa livens up the flavor of the halibut.

Halibut:

2 halibut filets, ⅓ lb or 155 g each

1 tbsp extra-virgin olive oil

Cherry tomatoes, for garnish

Quinoa:

½ cup (125 ml) **quinoa**

1 cup (250 ml) **water**

Pinch sea salt

½ cup (125 ml) **chayote, peeled and julienned**

1 large carrot, julienned

1 small leek, julienned

2 cloves garlic, minced

1 tbsp extra-virgin olive oil

Sea salt and fresh ground pepper, to taste

Salsa:

1 cup (250 ml) **cherry tomatoes, chopped**

2 tbsp fresh ginger, peeled and minced

2 tbsp chayote, peeled and minced

2 tbsp extra-virgin olive oil

1 tbsp apple cider vinegar

1 tbsp fresh dill, chopped

Sea salt and fresh ground pepper, to taste

Preheat oven to 375°F (190°C).

To prepare the vegetable quinoa, bring quinoa and salted water to a boil; reduce heat and simmer for 15 minutes or until all the water is absorbed and the quinoa is light and fluffy. In a large pan, heat oil over medium heat and sauté chayote, carrot, leek and garlic until tender. Stir in quinoa.

In the meantime, brown both sides of the halibut filets in olive oil then bake in the oven for 5 to 7 minutes or until done.

To make the salsa, thoroughly combine all the salsa ingredients in a bowl.

Place vegetable quinoa onto plates, arrange halibut over top, garnish with cherry tomatoes and salsa then serve.

Serves 2

cherry tomato

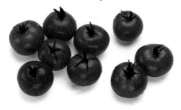

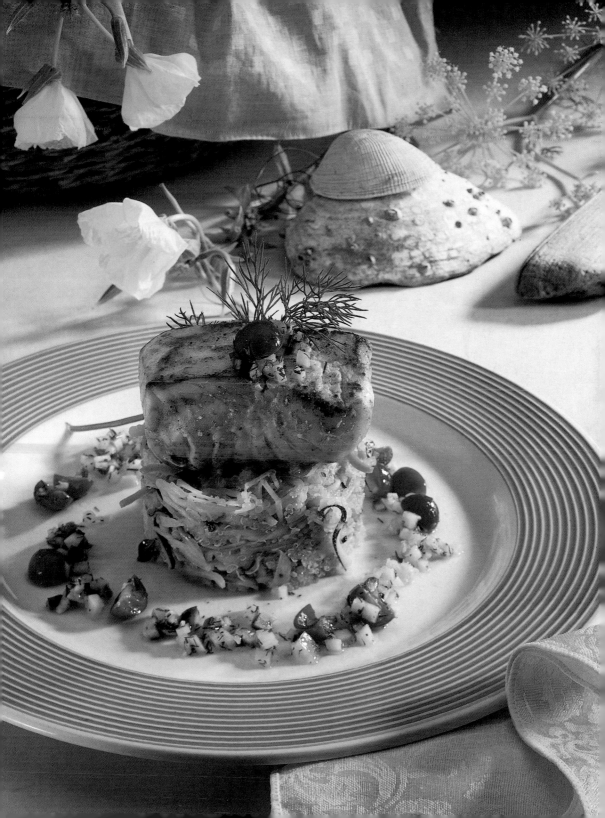

Zucchini Flower Stuffed with Brown Rice

Pluck the zucchini fresh from the garden with its flower still attached to make this unusual dish that pleases the eye as well as the taste buds. The intense color of the simple tomato sauce is so beautiful over top of the deep green and yellow of the zucchini and its flower, and it's easy to digest as well.

½ **cup** (125 ml) **onion, diced**

2 **cloves garlic, minced**

1 **tbsp ginger, minced**

1 **cup** (250 ml) **fresh green peas**

1 **small jalapeno pepper, finely diced** (optional)

½ **cup** (125 ml) **carrots, diced**

1 **cup** (250 ml) **short-grain brown rice** (or kamut or millet), **cooked**

1 **tbsp fresh dill, chopped**

Sea salt and freshly ground pepper, to taste

2 **tbsp extra-virgin olive oil**

1 **tbsp butter**

4 **small zucchinis with flowers**

onion

Sauce:

¼ **cup** (60 ml) **onion, chopped**

2 **medium-size ripe tomatoes, chopped**

2 **cloves garlic**

1 **tsp fresh dill, chopped**

1 **tbsp extra-virgin olive oil**

1 **tbsp butter**

Herbamare, to taste

In a pan, sauté onion, garlic and ginger in oil for 2 to 3 minutes until soft, then add peas, diced vegetables, rice, dill and seasonings; stir for 2 to 3 minutes longer. Add butter and stir to melt.

In the meantime, carefully snap off the stamen from the middle of each zucchini flower. Stuff the flower with the vegetable-rice mixture and twist the tips of the flower petals together. Carefully lay the zucchini in the steamer and steam for 5 to 6 minutes.

Meanwhile, make the sauce: purée onion, tomato and garlic in a food processor. Strain through a sieve into a saucepan and bring to a boil. Add olive oil and butter and simmer for 10 minutes until reduced by half. Stir in the dill and keep warm.

Place zucchini onto plates, pour sauce over top and serve.

Serves 2

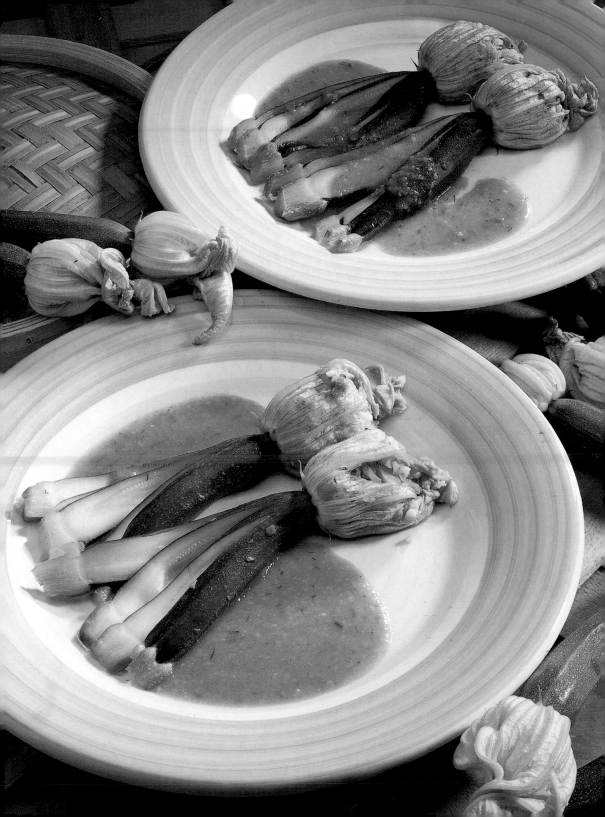

Vegetarian Shepherd's Pie

This very famous international dish is basically what the English make out of leftovers, but I'll gladly eat it because it's so nutritious and flavorful. The blanket of garlic mashed potato makes it a divine food.

2 lbs (1 kg) **russet potatoes**

3 cloves garlic, finely minced, divided

1 cup (250 ml) **kefir** (or natural buttermilk or yogurt)

1 cup (250 ml) **carrots, diced**

1 cup (250 ml) **celery, diced**

1 cup (250 ml) **onion, diced**

1 cup (250 ml) **zucchini, diced**

1 cup (250 ml) **eggplant, diced**

1 cup (250 ml) **tomatoes, diced**

2 tbsp extra-virgin olive oil

Dash paprika

Herbamare, to taste

1 tbsp fresh rosemary, chopped

Preheat the oven to 375°F (190°C).

Cook potatoes with skin in a pot of salted water for 20 to 25 minutes or until soft. Let cool then peel the potatoes and mash with a potato masher. Add 2 teaspoons of garlic and the kefir and mix well.

In the meantime, heat oil in a large pan over medium heat and sauté remaining garlic and vegetables for 5 to 7 minutes or until soft. Add spices and rosemary; cover and simmer for 5 minutes.

Pour vegetables into a baking dish then cover with mashed potato. Bake in the oven for 25 to 30 minutes or until the potato topping is golden brown.

Serves 2

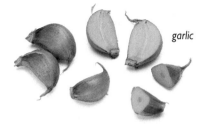

garlic

sources

Enzymatic Therapy
825 Challenger Drive
Green Bay, Wisconsin
54311-8328 USA

Enzymatic Therapy Canada Inc
Burnaby, BC
1-800-665-3414

Flora
7400 Fraser Park Drive
Burnaby BC V5J 5B9
604–436–6000
800–663–0617 (Western Canada)
800–387–7541 (Eastern Canada)

Naturade Inc
14370 Myford Rd, Suite 101
Irvine, CA 92606
Tel: 1-800-367-2880
Fax: 714-573-4818
International Fax: 714-573-4819
www.naturade.com

Natural Factors
3655 Bonneville Place
Burnaby, BC
V3N 4S9
1-800-663-8900

Omega Nutrition of Canada, Inc.
1924 Franklin Street
Vancouver BC V5L 1R2
604–253–4677
800–661–3529
www.omegaflo.com

Samra Health & Beauty, Inc
3000 S. Robertson Blvd.
Suite 420
Los Angeles, CA 90034
1-888-41 Samra
Fax: 310-202-8999
www.samra.com

Source Naturals, Inc
19 Janis Way, Scotts Valley, CA
95066
Tel:1-800-815-2333
Fax: 831-438-7410
Email: gavins@thresholdent.com
www.sourcenaturals.com

Remedies and supplements mentioned
in this book are available at quality
health food stores and nutrition centers.

First published in 2000 by
alive **books**
7436 Fraser Park Drive
Burnaby BC V5J 5B9
(604) 435–1919
1-800–661–0303

© 2000 by *alive* books

Book Design:
    Liza Novecoski
Artwork:
    Terence Yeung
    Raymond Cheung
Food Styling/Recipe Development:
    Fred Edrissi
Photography:
    Edmond Fong
    Siegfried Gursche
Photo Editing:
    Sabine Edrissi-Bredenbrock
Editing:
    Sandra Tonn

Canadian Cataloguing in
Publication Data

Babal CN, Ken
    Good Digestion

(*alive* natural health guides, 25
ISSN 1490-6503)
ISBN 1-55312-025-6

Printed in Canada

Revolutionary Health Books
alive Natural Health Guides

Each 64-page book focuses on a single subject, is written in easy-to-understand language and is lavishly illustrated with full color photographs.

New titles will be published every month.

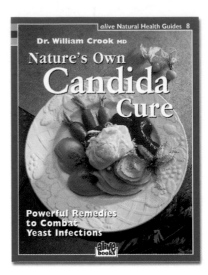

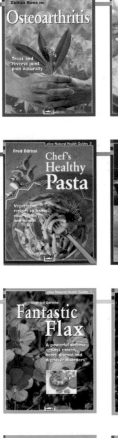
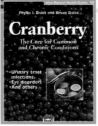
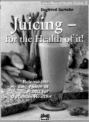
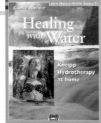